50 THING
BOOK SERIES
REVIEWS FROM READERS

I recently downloaded a couple of books from this series to read over the weekend thinking I would read just one or two. However, I so loved the books that I read all the six books I had downloaded in one go and ended up downloading a few more today. Written by different authors, the books offer practical advice on how you can perform or achieve certain goals in life, which in this case is how to have a better life.

The information is simple to digest and learn from, and is incredibly useful. There are also resources listed at the end of the book that you can use to get more information.

50 Things To Know To Have A Better Life: Self-Improvement Made Easy!

Author Dannii Cohen

This book is very helpful and provides simple tips on how to improve your everyday life. I found it to be useful in improving my overall attitude.

50 Things to Know For Your Mindfulness & Meditation Journey
Author Nina Edmondso

Quick read with 50 short and easy tips for what to think about before starting to homeschool.

50 Things to Know About Getting Started with Homeschool by Author Amanda Walton

I really enjoyed the voice of the narrator, she speaks in a soothing tone. The book is a really great reminder of things we might have known we could do during stressful times, but forgot over the years.

Author Harmony Hawaii

There is so much waste in our society today. Everyone should be forced to read this book. I know I am passing it on to my family.

50 Things to Know to Downsize Your Life: How To Downsize, Organize, And Get Back to Basics

Author Lisa Rusczyk Ed. D.

Great book to get you motivated and understand why you may be losing motivation. Great for that person who wants to start getting healthy, or just for you when you need motivation while having an established workout routine.

50 Things To Know To Stick With A Workout: Motivational Tips To Start The New You Today

Author Sarah Hughes

50 THINGS TO KNOW ABOUT BREAST CANCER

Written by A Survivor

Ronda K. Salazar

Cover designed by: Ivana Stamenkovic
Cover Image: https://pixabay.com/photos/forest-trail-
sunbeams-forest-path-2942477/

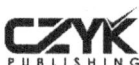

CZYK
PUBLISHING

CZYK Publishing Since 2011.
CZYKPublishing.com
50 Things to Know

Lock Haven, PA
All rights reserved.
ISBN: 9798455473197

50 THINGS TO KNOW ABOUT BREAST CANCER

BOOK DESCRIPTION

Do you have a friend or loved one who has breast cancer, and you are unsure of the best way to support them? Are you aware of the risk factors associated with developing breast cancer? If you knew of specific changes you could make today that would reduce the risk of breast cancer, would you put plans in place to make those changes? If you answered yes to any of these questions, then this book is for you.

50 Things To Know About Breast Cancer by Ronda K. Salazar offers an approach to discovering everything you need to know about breast cancer so you can be more proactive about your health or the health of a friend or loved one. Most books on breast cancer tell you all about the symptoms and what to expect during treatment. Although there's nothing wrong with that, they don't always provide good information on breast cancer awareness and early detection so you can potentially avoid getting breast cancer altogether. Based on knowledge from the world's leading experts and cancer organizations, Ronda takes the time to explain what breast cancer is, the different types of breast cancer and their symptoms, and the importance of early detection.

In these pages, you'll also discover some of the myths about breast cancer that often prevent women from getting their annual mammograms and checkups. You will gain some insights into what life is like living through a breast cancer diagnosis and ways to provide support for a friend or loved one facing breast cancer. This book will also help you recognize ways to be your own early detection advocate. So grab your copy of this book today. You'll be glad you did.

TABLE OF CONTENTS

DEDICATION

I dedicate this book to my very best friend, Howard, who held me up and cared for me when I literally couldn't lift a hand for myself. You are my rock, my foundation, and I am forever grateful to have you in my life. I know we will remain lifelong friends, and we have many more adventures to experience together.

To my Bugaboo Ori, everything I do is for my girl! I love you so much and am so proud of everything you have achieved already in your young life. You are and always will be my sunshine!

To my brother, Ron, who did what our family does best and immediately went into planning mode when I was too shocked and terrified to do anything myself. Thank you for always having my back.

For all my co-workers (you know who you all are), thank you for supporting me in a very traumatic time in my life. You all rallied together to care for me in ways that I didn't even know I needed. Picture Friday's will forever hold a special place in my heart. Thank you for lifting me up so effortlessly.

Finally, this book is for anyone who has been diagnosed with breast cancer. We are all at different stages of this journey and I honor each and every one of you. Through the facts and insights in this book, I hope to provide tools for everyone impacted by breast cancer.

ABOUT THE AUTHOR

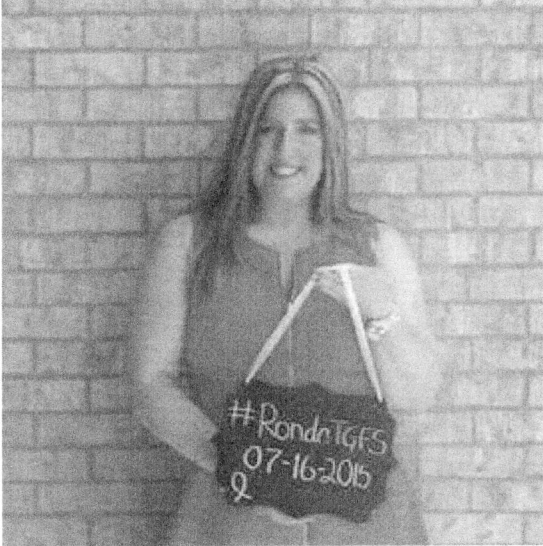

Photo by candracreative

Ronda K. Salazar is a breast cancer survivor. She was unexpectedly diagnosed in June of 2015 after getting her first mammogram at 46. Ronda was extremely fortunate as she caught her cancer very early. However, if she had elected to wait for another 2 to 3 months to get her first mammogram, her story today would have been much different.

Ronda chose to have a double mastectomy to rid her body of cancer. Her cancer was aggressive and had started spreading by the time she had surgery, only four weeks after her diagnosis. Ronda often shares with others that she "cheated cancer at its own game." Since she chose a double mastectomy, which was considered an aggressive and extreme surgery option, Ronda did not have to go through chemotherapy, radiation treatment, or long-term pill therapy. There are many side effects of those treatments, and Ronda was able to avoid those side effects altogether!

Ronda is extremely passionate about sharing her story. She openly shares her experience and hopes to help other women realize the importance of early detection and regular screening tests.

You can read all about Ronda's personal story and experience with breast cancer on her website at http://www.rondatgfs.com.

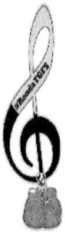

Ronda's Personal Logo and Hashtag (#RondaTGFS)

INTRODUCTION

"There can be life after breast cancer. The prerequisite is early detection."

Ann Jillian

C ancer is a scary disease that seems to come out of nowhere and turns life upside down. You may have a friend or a close relative with some type of cancer - it affects everyone either directly or indirectly - or perhaps you have been diagnosed with cancer yourself.

When I was diagnosed with breast cancer, I initially didn't know how to react or what to do. There isn't a checklist that tells us everything we have to do to survive cancer. There's no magic book, no secret sisterhood, no underground resources that can fix a cancer diagnosis. All we can do is to tackle it: learn everything we can about our type of cancer and lean on friends and loved ones for moral support. Most of all, we should be our own health advocates. We need to ask questions and challenge our doctors instead of taking what they say and running with it. Cancer treatment is not a one-size-fits-all solution, so doctors must think through everything about our specific diagnosis and situation.

I was very fortunate because I discovered I had breast cancer when it was still in the early stages. As a result, I did not require radiation, chemotherapy, or a long-term pill regimen. Instead, I elected to have a double mastectomy. I wanted to remove as much breast tissue as possible from my body to minimize the chances of the big "C" ever coming back to attack my breasts again.

At this present time, while I am writing this book, I am almost six years cancer-free. I have spent countless hours fundraising for non-profit breast cancer awareness and research organizations. I have spoken at several awareness events. I even created an instrumental CD of original piano compositions to tell my story. I want to make a difference in this world and help other women know that when you get your boobs squished for that annual mammogram, you're doing it to save those boobs. Early detection is crucial because it can save your life. It saved mine.

I have divided this book into four sections. In the first section, I offer fact-based information about breast cancer from the world's leading experts and cancer organizations as well as through my personal experiences. The second section tackles some of the myths about breast cancer that prevent women from getting the proper early detection screening tests. In the third section, I share details about my own experience living with breast cancer. I include some extremely personal and intimate details about what happens to a woman, both physically and psychologically, after hearing a breast cancer diagnosis and having a mastectomy. Finally, in the last section, I share information about supporting a friend or loved one diagnosed with breast cancer.

Whether you are facing breast cancer yourself or supporting a friend or loved one going through breast cancer, I hope that this book gives you the strength and courage to face it head-on and with compassion and empathy. No one should ever have to face a breast cancer diagnosis alone.

FACTS ABOUT BREAST CANCER

1. WHAT IS BREAST CANCER?

Breast Cancer is a type of cancer that forms when cells in the breast begin to develop and grow out of control abnormally. Cancer occurs as a result of cell mutations or abnormal changes to the underlying cell structure.

The anatomy of a breast consists of a nipple, lobules, ducts, fat and connective tissue. The lobules are the milk-producing glands within the breast. The ducts are the passages that drain the milk from the lobules to the nipples. The formation of cell mutation typically starts in the lobules or ducts, and in rare instances, it can begin in the nipple.

Any type of cancer can spread (metastasize) outside of the originating body part or organ. The metastasis begins when malignant cells break off from the original tumor or mass and enter the blood vessels or the lymph nodes. Cancer cells can travel through the blood or the lymphatic system and spread to distant areas of the body. Once the cancer cells spread, the necessary treatment to eradicate the cancer cells becomes more serious and complex. This alone is a critical reason why early detection is so important with any type of cancer.

2. WHO CAN GET BREAST CANCER?

Although it is widely thought that women are the only people at risk, men can also get breast cancer. Men account for about 1% of all breast cancer diagnoses in the United States.[1]

During puberty, boys and girls develop a few ducts around the nipples. After puberty, as girls begin to grow, they continue to produce female hormones, which cause the ducts and lobules to form in the girls' breasts. Boys have low levels of female hormones after puberty and do not see significant growth of breast tissue.

That doesn't mean that men have no risk of breast cancer, however. They still have breast tissue, and cells can mutate in any part of the body to create cancerous tumors.

Breast cancer awareness is the key! It can be somewhat embarrassing for a man diagnosed with

---

[1]Centers for Disease Control and Prevention (2020). 'Breast Cancer in Men', *Centers for Disease Control and Prevention.* Retrieved from https://www.cdc.gov/cancer/breast/men/index.htm.

breast cancer, as most people consider this a type of cancer that can only affect women. However, it is imperative men pay attention to any unexpected changes in their chest area. If a tumor does form, early detection will make the treatment and prognosis more promising.

3. BREAST CANCER STATISTICS

Breast cancer is the second most common cancer for women in the United States, with skin cancer being the most common. As of 2021, one in eight women (13%) can expect to be diagnosed with breast cancer at some time in their lifetime.[2] This statistic is staggering if you stop to consider what that means.

Next time you sit in a class at school, a training course or workshop, church, movie theater, or restaurant, take a look around you. Count the number of women that you see. If there are forty women, then five women in that group will get breast cancer at

---

[2] The American Cancer Society medical and editorial content team (2021). 'How Common Is Breast Cancer?', *American Cancer Society*. Retrieved from https://www.cancer.org/cancer/breast-cancer/about/how-common-is-breast-cancer.html.

some point in their life. It could be someone sitting right next to you! That thought is extremely sobering!

On a positive note, there are currently about 3.8 million breast cancer survivors in the United States alone.[3] In addition, treatments are becoming more targeted and sophisticated, and death rates are beginning to decline, especially for women who get breast cancer after 50.

4. BREAST CANCER RISK FACTORS YOU CAN CONTROL

Do you have specific risk factors associated with developing breast cancer? Having a risk factor does not automatically mean that you will get breast cancer, but the chances of being diagnosed in your lifetime do increase significantly.

Some of the risks associated with breast cancer are things you can control and change:[4]

---

[3] Centers for Disease Control and Prevention (2020). 'What Are the Risk Factors for Breast Cancer?', *Centers for Disease Control and Prevention.* Retrieved from https://www.cdc.gov/cancer/breast/basic_info/risk_factors.htm.

[4] The American Cancer Society medical and editorial content team (2021). 'How Common Is Breast Cancer?', *American Cancer Society.* Retrieved from https://www.cancer.org/cancer/breast-cancer/about/how-

- <u>Little physical activity</u> - It is imperative to stay active, especially as you begin to get older. The body needs physical exertion to remain strong, which gives you a better chance of fighting off disease and illness.
- <u>Overweight</u> - If you are overweight, this places more stress on your internal organs. Your body loses its ability to fight off infection and combat cell mutations.
- <u>First pregnancy after 30</u> - Some studies show that if you have your first pregnancy after 30, it can increase the risk of getting breast cancer.
- <u>Hormone replacement therapy</u> - Estrogen and progesterone hormone therapy can reduce the symptoms of menopause. However, when used for more than five years, some forms can increase the chances of getting breast cancer.
- <u>Drinking alcohol</u> - There have been studies performed that indicate the more alcohol a woman drinks directly increases the woman's risk for breast cancer.
- <u>Smoking</u> - Although smoking is often linked to lung cancer, it can also increase the risk for breast cancer.

---

common-is-breast-cancer.html.

5. BREAST CANCER RISK FACTORS YOU CANNOT CONTROL

There are many risk factors associated with breast cancer that you cannot control or change. These factors are more severe and should be paid close attention to, especially if any of them are true for you:[5]

- <u>Getting older</u> - There is an increased risk of developing breast cancer with age.
- <u>Genetic mutations</u> - Women who have the BRCA gene mutation have a significantly higher risk of getting breast cancer than women who do not have a mutation.[6]
- <u>Never having a full-term pregnancy</u> - Women who never get pregnant or never carry a pregnancy to term are at a higher risk of getting breast cancer in their lifetime.

---

[5] Centers for Disease Control and Prevention (2020). 'What Are the Risk Factors for Breast Cancer?', *Centers for Disease Control and Prevention.* Retrieved from https://www.cdc.gov/cancer/breast/basic_info/risk_factors.htm.

[6] Having the BRCA gene does not mean a woman will absolutely get breast cancer. However, there is a much higher chance it can occur. About 50% of the women with a BRCA gene mutation will get breast cancer by the time they are 70 years old. Women who have the BRCA gene mutation should talk with their doctor about screening and other ways to reduce their risk.

- <u>Dense breasts</u> - Women with dense breasts may need to use different screening methods such as 3D mammograms and ultrasounds. These types of tests are more likely to detect cancer cells in dense breast tissue.
- <u>Family history of breast cancer</u> - If you have a family history of breast cancer, you are more at risk for developing breast cancer.[7]
- <u>Radiation therapy</u> - There is a higher than average risk of developing breast cancer if before the age of 30 you had any radiation therapy to the chest for something other than breast cancer.

Making changes to reduce risks you can control is a healthy first step in fighting breast cancer.

---

[7] If you have one close relative with breast cancer (sister, mother, or daughter), you double your risk for developing breast cancer. If you have two close relatives, your risk is five times higher than average. Know your family history and understand your risks. Be sure to talk with your doctor if you have any history of breast cancer in your family.

6. TYPES OF BREAST CANCER

There are two general types of breast cancer: non-invasive and invasive. In addition, there are more specific types of breast cancer within each of these categories, depending on the types of affected breast cells.

Non-invasive breast cancer is referred to as "in situ," which means "situated in the original place." This type of breast cancer has not spread outside of the milk ducts or lobules.

Invasive breast cancer is referred to as "infiltrating" breast cancer. Invasive breast cancer describes any breast cancer that has spread outside of the milk ducts or lobules and into the surrounding breast tissue.

7. TYPES OF NON-INVASIVE BREAST CANCER

There are two main types of non-invasive breast cancer:[8]

- <u>Ductal Carcinoma In Situ (DCIS)</u> is a type of cancer that starts in the milk ducts and has not spread into the rest of the breast tissue.
- <u>Lobular Carcinoma in Situ (LCIS)</u> is not technically considered a form of cancer. Instead, it is viewed as a change in the breast. Cells that resemble cancer cells can grow inside the lobules. It is crucial to have regular checkups as this may put you at an increased risk of developing breast cancer later.

When I was first diagnosed with breast cancer, my doctor told me that I had DCIS. I had no idea what that even meant. It sounded like a foreign language to me. However, after doing some research, I realized that DCIS is a type of non-invasive breast cancer, and I was extremely fortunate because DCIS is very treatable and contained.

---

[8] Maurie Markman, MD, President, Medicine & Science at CTCA (2021). 'Breast cancer types', *Cancer Treatment Centers of America.* Retrieved from https://www.cancercenter.com/cancer-types/breast-cancer/types.

8. TYPES OF INVASIVE BREAST CANCER

If you recall, invasive breast cancer means that the cancer cells have "invaded" surrounding areas of the breast tissue outside of the duct. As a result, the cancer cells have spread outside of the originating site or location. There are many types of invasive breast cancer:[9]

- Invasive Ductal Carcinoma (IDC) - This is the most common type of breast cancer and represents approximately 80% of all breast cancer types. This type of cancer starts in the cells that line the milk ducts in the breast. As cancer cells begin to spread, the cancer cells break through the wall of the milk duct and into the surrounding tissue.
- Invasive Lobular Carcinoma (ILS) - This type of invasive breast cancer is similar to IDC, except it starts in the milk-producing glands (lobules). ILS is harder to detect on

---

[9] Maurie Markman, MD, President, Medicine & Science at CTCA (2021). 'Breast cancer types', *Cancer Treatment Centers of America.* Retrieved from https://www.cancercenter.com/cancer-types/breast-cancer/types.

mammograms, and unlike other breast cancers, there is a 20% chance that if one breast has ILS, the other breast will also be infected.

- Inflammatory Breast Cancer (IBC) - Inflammatory breast cancer is extremely rare and represents approximately 5% of all breast cancers. The symptoms of IBC are much different from other types of breast cancer. With IBC, the symptoms are inflammation, redness, and swelling on any area of the breast. These symptoms occur because cancer cells block the lymph vessels that restrict normal circulatory system functions.
- Paget's Disease of the Breast - This is a rare form of breast cancer often accompanied by ductal carcinoma (either in situ or invasive). This disease starts on the nipple itself and extends out into the areola.
- Angiosarcoma of the Breast - This type of breast cancer begins in the blood or lymphatic vessels within the breast. Although angiosarcoma of the breast is not common, it is aggressive and spreads quickly.

9. SYMPTOMS OF BREAST CANCER

Before I was diagnosed with breast cancer, I always thought that feeling a lump in your breast was the only indication that you might have breast cancer. I didn't realize other symptoms exist that you cannot see with the naked eye or feel by touch.

It is crucial to be aware of other symptoms that can be a possible sign of breast cancer, as these are early indicators that can help save your life. Here are some symptoms in addition to lumps that can be a warning sign for breast cancer:[10]

- Nipple discharge or bleeding
- Nipple pain
- Redness or swelling
- Nipple turning inward
- An increase in the size or shape of the breast
- Irritated or itchy breasts
- Peeling or flaking of the nipple skin
- Pitting or dimpling of the breast skin

---

[10] The American Cancer Society medical and editorial content team (2019). 'Breast Cancer Signs and Symptoms', *American Cancer Society.* Retrieved from https://www.cancer.org/cancer/breast-cancer/about/breast-cancer-signs-and-symptoms.html.

Some types of breast cancer do not have outwardly visible symptoms but have other characteristics that screening tests can detect:

- <u>Microcalcification</u> - This is an early warning sign for DCIS. It is a grouping of small "dots" that are visible only on a mammogram.[11]
- <u>Swollen lymph nodes</u> - Swollen lymph nodes are one of the critical indicators for Inflammatory Breast Cancer. These can appear under the arm or above the collarbone.

[11] When I had my first mammogram at the age of 46, the x-ray results showed a small collection of "dots" or microcalcification. At first, the Radiologist told me that only 20% of microcalcification ends up being cancerous. So the initial recommendation from the Radiologist was to "wait" and get another mammogram in six months to see if the area had gotten larger.

Waiting seemed like such a huge risk to me. There was a 1 in 5 chance that I had cancer, but I was supposed to wait for six months and get another test to see if it had started to spread! That was so unbelievable to me. So I insisted on having a biopsy. I was fortunate that I made that decision because I was the 1 in 5 statistical number. The "dots" on my mammogram were cancer cells.

Early detection is critical when it comes to the discovery of breast cancer. Know the symptoms that can be early indicators of breast cancer. Never be afraid or timid about challenging the recommendations of a radiologist or doctor when they review your screening test results. I questioned my Radiologist's recommendation, and it saved my life!

10. HOW IS BREAST CANCER DETECTED?

A mammogram is one of the most common methods for detecting potential cancer cells within the breast. However, it is also possible to detect a potential problem by feeling a lump or seeing a visual change in the shape or color of the breast.

By the time a lump is detected, the chances of cancer spreading outside of the breast tissue are extremely high. Getting regular mammograms is vital to ensure early detection of breast cancer cells before those cells form a lump that you can feel.

There are many other types of tests used to detect the presence of breast cancer. These tests are designated as either screening tests or diagnostic tests.

11. SCREENING TESTS VERSUS DIAGNOSTIC TESTS

Medical professionals perform screening tests as a proactive method for finding breast cancer in people who do not show any known symptoms. When you have a screening test performed on you, this is a direct action to take control of your health. If the test results indicate the presence of cancer-like cells, you have utilized early detection to diagnose a disease before the presence of external symptoms.

On the other hand, doctors utilize diagnostic tests to confirm a suspected breast cancer diagnosis obtained from a screening test. There are two types of diagnostic tests: invasive and non-invasive.

Invasive diagnostic testing involves entering the body or puncturing the skin. For example, a diagnostic biopsy test involves taking a sample of the affected area using a long needle. A biopsy can also be performed by surgically removing a small section of the infected area.

Non-invasive diagnostic testing is performed on the exterior of the body without breaking the skin. Examples of these types of tests include ultrasounds and diagnostic imaging tools.

12. RECOMMENDED GUIDELINES FOR BREAST CANCER SCREENING

The American Cancer Society is a non-profit organization with a mission to rid the world of cancer. They are a well-respected entity, and their guidelines for screening are considered the most reliable and trustworthy. They provide recommendations based on research, science, data, and facts.

According to the American Cancer Society, women without high-risk factors should use the following guidelines for breast cancer screening:[12]

- <u>Women ages 40 to 44</u> should have the choice to start annual mammogram screening if so desired.
- <u>Women between the ages of 45 and 54</u> should get a mammogram every year.
- <u>Women 55 and older</u> can continue with annual screening, or they may switch to mammograms every two years.

Women at a higher risk for breast cancer should consult with their doctor to determine the appropriate type and frequency of breast cancer screening.

13. BENIGN VERSUS MALIGNANT TUMORS

[12] The American Cancer Society medical and editorial content team (2021). 'American Cancer Society Recommendations for the Early Detection of Breast Cancer', *American Cancer Society*. Retrieved from https://www.cancer.org/cancer/breast-cancer/screening-tests-and-early-detection/american-cancer-society-recommendations-for-the-early-detection-of-breast-cancer.html.

It is important to remember that not all lumps or tumors are cancerous. If a tumor is considered non-cancerous, it is referred to as a "benign tumor." Most benign tumors are harmless unless they are pressing up against or interfering with the function of a specific organ, muscle, or nerve in the body. If a tumor or collection of cells is designated as cancerous, it is called a "malignant tumor."

14. GENETICS AND BREAST CANCER

There are two gene mutations, BRCA1 and BRCA2, linked to a higher risk of developing breast cancer and ovarian cancer. Since these genes carry hereditary information, any mutations of those genes get passed from parent to child. As a result, it's essential to know your family history. For example, if your mother, sister, or aunt has a history of breast cancer, genetic testing may help determine if you have either of the BRCA gene mutations.

If you have one of the gene mutations, keep in mind that this does not mean you will get breast cancer in your lifetime. However, it is a crucial warning sign that indicates an oncologist should closely monitor your health. In addition, it is essential to start screening tests at a younger age since early detection of breast cancer provides a better long-term prognosis.

When I first got my cancer diagnosis, I decided to have genetic testing performed. It can be a critical piece of information to have when deciding on the type of breast cancer treatment you need.

15. STAGES OF BREAST CANCER

There are different systems used to define the stages of breast cancer. The determination of the stage of breast cancer can be clinical or pathological. Clinical staging is based on screening and diagnostic tests performed before surgery.

Pathological staging is based on test results and discoveries during surgery when removing breast tissue and lymph nodes. In general, pathological staging provides the most details regarding the progression of the disease.

The most common system used for describing the stage of breast cancer is the TNM system defined by the American Joint Committee on Cancer. The results obtained by using the TNM system combined with other factors specific to the type of cancer determine the overall cancer stage.

Most people are more familiar with the cancer stage grouping or numerical staging system, usually represented as 0, I, II, III, or IV. The lower the number, the less the cancer cells have spread. Some of these numbered stages also have subcategories: letter designations of A, B, or C. The earlier the letter is in the alphabet, the less the cancer has spread. The subcategory provides additional details regarding the progression of that particular breast cancer stage.

16. KEY INFORMATION USED TO DETERMINE THE STAGE

A medical professional uses several pieces of information to determine the stage of breast cancer in a patient accurately.[13] Each piece of information is critical for determining the stage, the prognosis, and the treatment plan. Identifying the specific cancer stage is a complex challenge, and as doctors and

[13] Maurie Markman, MD, President, Medicine & Science at CTCA (2021). 'Breast cancer stages', *Cancer Treatment Centers of America.* Retrieved from https://www.cancercenter.com/cancer-types/breast-cancer/stages.

researchers learn more about cancer, the methods for determining the stage may change slightly over time. Doctors and researchers continually refine the staging process to provide more specific and granular details about a particular type of cancer.

- TNM System - T Category: Overall size of the tumor
- TNM System - N Category: Number of lymph nodes affected
- TNM System - M Category: Presence and extent of metastasis
- Estrogen Receptor Status: Presence of estrogen receptor in cancer cells
- Progesterone Receptor Status: Presence of progesterone receptor in cancer cells
- HER2 Status: How much of the HER2 protein is present in the cells
- Cancer Grade: The appearance of the cancer cells compared to normal cells

On June 19, 2015, I was diagnosed with breast cancer. My Radiologist used clinical staging to define my diagnosis, Stage 0 (DCIS). On July 16, 2015, I had a total mastectomy of my right breast (the infected breast) and a prophylactic mastectomy of my left breast. My doctor sent samples of my breast tissue to a lab for final testing. My pathological staging designation changed to Stage 1A based on the examination of my physical breast tissue.

In the following sections, I will explain each critical piece of information used to deterzmine the breast cancer stage.

17. TNM SYSTEM

With the TNM system, there are three main categories or characteristics used to evaluate breast cancer:

- <u>T (tumor) category</u>: This describes the primary or original tumor and associated biomarkers.
- <u>N (node) category</u>: This indicates whether or not lymph nodes are affected, which means cancer has started to spread.
- <u>M (metastasis) category</u>: This category defines whether cancer has spread or metastasized to more distant areas of the body.

18. TNM SYSTEM - T CATEGORY

The primary tumor location is the spot in the body where cancer cells first started. When assigning the T category stage, doctors use three key factors: the primary tumor size, specific location, and determination of whether it has spread to nearby areas.

The T category consists of a letter and a number designation:[14]

- **TX**: This means no information is available, or the primary tumor cannot be evaluated and measured.
- **T0**: This assignment indicates there is no evidence of a primary tumor in the breast.
- **T1, T, T3, T4**: This category references the size of the primary tumor. The higher the number, the larger the tumor or the more the tumor has spread into nearby tissue.

---

[14] National Cancer Institute (2015). 'Cancer Staging', *National Cancer Institute.* Retrieved from https://www.cancer.gov/about-cancer/diagnosis-staging/staging.

19. TNM SYSTEM - N CATEGORY

One of the main tests performed during surgery is a biopsy and removal of the sentinel lymph node.[15] The surgeon will evaluate the size of the tumor and the extent of the spread of cancer cells into nearby tissue. Based on findings, the surgeon may remove additional lymph nodes to determine the extent of the possible spread of cancer outside of the breast.

The N category is defined by a letter and a number:[16]

- **NX**:- This means that it is impossible to measure or determine if cancer exists in nearby lymph nodes.
- **N0**: Lymph nodes have been tested, and there is no presence of cancer. This is an indication that cancer has likely not spread outside of the breast tissue.
- **N1, N2, N3**: This refers to the number of lymph nodes that contain cancer cells and

---

[15] The sentinel lymph node is the very first lymph node underneath the arm (in the armpit) and is typically the first lymph node within a group of nodes that cancer cells will pass through from the primary tumor in the breast.

[16] National Cancer Institute (2015). 'Cancer Staging', *National Cancer Institute.* Retrieved from https://www.cancer.gov/about-cancer/diagnosis-staging/staging.

their location. The higher the number, the more lymph nodes that are affected.

20. TNM SYSTEM - M CATEGORY

The M category measures the extent of metastasis, if applicable. The M category is defined as one of the following:[17]

- **MX**: This means that the surgeon cannot determine the presence of metastasis.
- **M0**: This category designation means the surgeon has confirmed that cancer has not spread to other parts of the body.
- **M1**: This designation means cancer has spread to other parts of the body.

---

[17] National Cancer Institute (2015). 'Cancer Staging', *National Cancer Institute.* Retrieved from https://www.cancer.gov/about-cancer/diagnosis-staging/staging.

21. HORMONE RECEPTOR STATUS

There are specific types of proteins within cancer cells known as receptors, and they can attach themselves to certain substances within the blood. Therefore, the hormone receptor status is a crucial piece of information used to determine the stage of breast cancer and overall cancer treatment strategy.

The two hormone receptors known to fuel breast cancer growth are estrogen and progesterone receptors. Normal breast cells and some cancer cells have receptors that attach to estrogen and progesterone. Therefore, these cells depend on these hormones to grow.[18]

Suppose the cancer cells have one or both of the hormone receptors. Doctors prescribe specific drugs to target these hormones. Those drugs will lower the hormone levels or stop the hormones from attaching to and acting on breast cancer cells.

---

[18] Breastcancer.org (2020). 'Hormone Receptor Status', *Breastcancer.org.* Retrieved from https://www.breastcancer.org/symptoms/diagnosis/hormone_status.

22. ESTROGEN AND PROGESTERONE RECEPTOR STATUS DESIGNATIONS

Breast cancer cells can have only estrogen receptors, only progesterone receptors, or both receptors. Doctors perform tests to determine the presence of these receptors and will then assign one of the following designations:[19]

- **ER-positive or ER+**: This designation indicates if the breast cancer cells have estrogen receptors.
- **PR-positive or PR+**: Breast cancer cells with progesterone receptors use this designation.
- **Hormone receptor-positive or HR+**: If the cancer cells have one or both of the hormone receptors, then the cancer may be referred to using this designation.
- **Hormone receptor-negative or HR-**: This status applies to cancer cells that do not have estrogen or progesterone receptors.

---

[19] The American Cancer Society medical and editorial content team (2019). 'Breast Cancer Hormone Receptor Status', *American Cancer Society.* Retrieved from https://www.cancer.org/cancer/breast-cancer/understanding-a-breast-cancer-diagnosis/breast-cancer-hormone-receptor-status.html.

23. HER2 STATUS

HER2 is a type of protein that exists in all breast cells. It stands for "human epidermal growth factor 2." This is a growth-promoting protein, which means it can increase the speed at which the cancer cells grow if too much of the protein exists in the cells.[20] As a result, the cancer cells will spread faster than other breast cancers. On a positive note, some drugs specifically target the HER2 protein to inhibit the growth of those cancer cells.

Some breast cancer cases have cells without estrogen receptors, progesterone receptors, or a high amount of HER2 receptors. These particular cases are called "triple-negative." However, if the cancer cells have all three of these receptors, then the term "triple-positive" is used to describe the cancer.

---

[20] Karthik Giridhar, M.D. (2020). 'HER2-positive breast cancer: What is it?', *Mayo Clinic*. Retrieved from https://www.mayoclinic.org/breast-cancer/expert-answers/faq-20058066.

24. BREAST CANCER GRADE

Once cancer cells are removed from the breast, they are analyzed to determine how much they look like <u>normal</u> cells. The grade, along with other factors previously described, is used to help determine treatment and prognosis. There are three possible grades: 1, 2, and 3.[21]

A lower grade number, such as 1, usually is an indicator that the cancer is growing slowly. With a higher grade number such as 3, the cancer cells are faster-growing. A higher grade number indicates that the cancer cells can spread more easily and quickly to other parts of the body.

---

[21] The American Cancer Society medical and editorial content team (2019). 'Breast Cancer Grades', *American Cancer Society.* Retrieved from https://www.cancer.org/cancer/breast-cancer/understanding-a-breast-cancer-diagnosis/breast-cancer-grades.html.

25. BREAST CANCER TREATMENT OPTIONS

Several types of treatment are available for breast cancer patients. The type of treatment(s) needed is very dependent on the breast cancer stage and type of breast cancer.

Some of the standard treatments used include:[22]

- Surgery
- Radiation therapy
- Chemotherapy
- Hormone therapy
- Targeted drug therapy
- Immunotherapy

When treating breast cancer, a patient may require a single treatment option or a combination of multiple treatments. Each treatment option has pros and cons as well as potential side effects. If you are facing a breast cancer diagnosis, it is critical that you fully understand and discuss all treatment options with your doctor before making a decision.

---

[22] Centers for Disease Control and Prevention (2020). 'How Is Breast Cancer Treated?', *Centers for Disease Control and Prevention.* Retrieved from https://www.cdc.gov/cancer/breast/basic_info/treatment.htm.

37

26. BREAST CANCER TREATMENT - SURGERY

When I was diagnosed with breast cancer in my right breast, I honestly felt like my world had been completely shattered. It was a very unexpected diagnosis. I met with a breast surgeon who laid out all the possible options for me based on my current breast cancer stage, Stage 0 (DCIS).

I had several treatment options available to me. The breast surgeon described them to me in the following order, with her recommended option listed first:

1. The breast surgeon recommended what is called a <u>lumpectomy</u> or <u>breast-conserving surgery</u>.[23]

2. The next recommended option for me was a <u>total mastectomy</u>[24] of my right (affected)

---

[23] A <u>lumpectomy</u> or <u>breast-conserving surgery</u> is a procedure that involves surgically removing just the part of the breast and surrounding tissue that contains the cancer cells. It leaves the remaining breast tissue and breast structure intact, thus conserving the breast. It's literally taking a scoop out of the breast and then stitching it together to close the hole left behind.

[24] A <u>total mastectomy</u> involves surgically removing the entire breast infected with cancer, including the breast tissue and some of the skin.

breast and a <u>prophylactic mastectomy</u>[25] of my left breast.

3. The last option was a <u>nipple-sparing mastectomy</u>,[26] which was not possible for me due to the location of my cancer cells.

Women who choose to have a mastectomy will often also elect to have breast reconstruction surgery. The surgery rebuilds the shape of the breast using implants or a patient's own non-breast tissue. Reconstruction surgery can be performed at the time of the mastectomy or at a later time.

As you can tell, there are many options that a woman has to think through when facing a breast cancer diagnosis. After weighing all my options out very carefully, I finally decided that I wanted a bilateral mastectomy: a total mastectomy on my right breast (infected with cancer) and a prophylactic mastectomy on the left side (for peace of mind). I

---

[25] A <u>prophylactic mastectomy</u> involves removing a non-infected breast to reduce the risk of developing breast cancer in that breast. This type of surgery is not medically necessary, but many women choose to do this for peace of mind.

[26] A <u>nipple-sparing mastectomy</u> is a surgical procedure that does not involve removing the nipple or the areola. This surgical option saves most of the breast skin, as well. This option is not always viable for a woman with breast cancer. It depends on the size of the tumor and cells and the location of the cancer cells.

wanted to rid my body of as much breast tissue as possible, so I wouldn't continually worry about whether the cancer was coming back.[27]

27. BREAST CANCER TREATMENT - RADIATION THERAPY

Radiation therapy is typically used after having breast-conserving surgery. In some cases, it may be performed prior to surgery to help shrink tumors. Radiation therapy uses high-energy x-rays to target cancer cells and kill them or prevent them from growing larger. Radiation can be applied externally, using a machine outside of the body to target cancer

[27] When I went to see my oncologist after my double mastectomy, he told me that it was really not necessary for me to undergo any chemotherapy or hormone therapy. He based his explanation on the data evidence and the particular stage of my breast cancer, which was Stage 1A. In my case, since I had elected to use surgery to remove most of my breast tissue, the odds of recurrence were less than 1%.

My oncologist continued to explain that the side effects from any additional chemotherapy or hormone therapy would be far worse than the benefits of trying to reduce a less than 1% chance of cancer coming back. In addition, the hormone therapy would force me into menopause, which meant hot flashes and possibly other side effects. I was fortunate since I didn't require treatments with significant visual and physical side effects.

cells. It can also be applied internally using a sealed radioactive substance placed near the cancer cells.[28]

28. BREAST CANCER TREATMENT - CHEMOTHERAPY

Chemotherapy is one of the most common treatment options for breast cancer. It uses one or more anti-cancer drugs to eradicate the cancer cells, reduce symptoms or prolong life. Chemotherapy treatment can target a specific area within the body or be introduced into the blood to reach all cancer cells throughout the body.

Chemotherapy can be delivered in multiple ways, depending on the type of treatment that is required. For example, it can be given in pill form, through an intravenous drip, as a shot or injection, or even topically. In some cases, chemotherapy may be given prior to a surgical treatment option to shrink existing cancer tumors.

---

[28] The American Cancer Society medical and editorial content team (2019). 'Radiation for Breast Cancer', *American Cancer Society.* Retrieved from https://www.cancer.org/cancer/breast-cancer/treatment/radiation-for-breast-cancer.html.

Chemotherapy is often given on a routine schedule or in intervals referred to as cycles. A single cycle may consist of multiple drugs given at a single time. A recovery period allows the drugs to work and provides time for the normal cells to recover from the side effects of the chemotherapy. This recovery period can be several days or several weeks.

Chemotherapy often has significant side effects. Loss of hair is a common side effect, but other side effects can be more damaging to internal organs. It also tends to deplete the immune system, resulting in fatigue, nausea, and other side effects that are not so pleasant.[29]

---

[29] The American Cancer Society medical and editorial content team (2019). 'Chemotherapy for Breast Cancer', *American Cancer Society*. Retrieved from https://www.cancer.org/cancer/breast-cancer/treatment/chemotherapy-for-breast-cancer.html.

29. BREAST CANCER TREATMENT - HORMONE THERAPY

Oncologists use hormone therapy for breast cancer that is hormone receptor-positive. It is typically an oral pill that the patient must take for several years after completing the primary treatment. The drugs used in hormone therapy block hormones from attaching to the estrogen and progesterone receptors, thus reducing the chances of cancer cell growth.

30. BREAST CANCER TREATMENT - TARGETED DRUG THERAPY

Doctors use targeted drug therapy to specifically target the changes in cells that cause cancer to grow. In addition, researchers are discovering more ways to inhibit specific cell growth characteristics. Targeted drug therapy is very similar to chemotherapy as the drugs are introduced into the bloodstream to reach and treat all areas of the body.[30]

---

[30] The American Cancer Society medical and editorial content team (2021). 'Targeted Drug Therapy for Breast Cancer', *American Cancer Society.* Retrieved from https://www.cancer.org/cancer/breast-cancer/treatment/targeted-

31. BREAST CANCER TREATMENT - IMMUNOTHERAPY

Immunotherapy is also known as immuno-oncology or biological therapy. This type of cancer treatment specifically uses the body's immune system to recognize and attack cancer cells. It can activate or suppress the immune system as needed to prevent the growth and spread of cancer cells. The tricky part of immunotherapy is that it must prevent the immune system from also attacking normal cells.[31]

---

therapy-for-breast-cancer.html.

[31] The American Cancer Society medical and editorial content team (2020). 'Immunotherapy for Breast Cancer', *American Cancer Society*. Retrieved from https://www.cancer.org/cancer/breast-cancer/treatment/immunotherapy.html.

BREAST CANCER MYTHS

32. BREAKING THE MYTH CYCLE

There are many misperceptions about breast cancer. Unfortunately, some of these incorrect understandings and myths prevent women from getting regular mammograms or other screening tests critical for female health and wellness.

We have so much information at our fingertips today with internet resources, social media, blogs, television, and streaming services. It is easy for anyone with an opinion to write an article or create a blog post to provide their perspective on cancer treatments and options. However, we need to recognize that a stated opinion is not necessarily a proven fact. When it comes to our health and well-being, we must be able to distinguish between a myth and a fact before placing all our trust in something.

My family has a history of various types of cancer. I have lost some relatives due to cancer, and as a result, I developed a fear of the unknown. If I don't know there is a problem, it seems logical that the problem doesn't exist. Therefore, I waited until I was 46 to get my first mammogram because I was terrified of finding out the results. Guidelines at the time recommended that annual mammograms start when a woman reaches the age of 40. I waited six years because I was afraid of finding something. It's not logical reasoning, but it is the reality that I had created for myself.

After I was diagnosed with breast cancer, I realized many women had the same kind of fear as I did. The fear of getting the results is a strong deterrent for having annual screening tests performed. There are also many myths about breast cancer causes and treatments that are not true. I will share some of these myths with you in future sections.

If you only remember one thing from this book, please remember this: **Breast cancer is very treatable when discovered early.** Early detection alone is one of the reasons I am writing this book. I want women (and men) to recognize that early detection of breast cancer is extremely important and can save your life. The sooner breast cancer is detected, the less chance it has to spread or metastasize in distant organs.

In the following few sections, I will provide you with facts that will dispel some of the more common breast cancer myths.

33. MYTH #1: NO FAMILY HISTORY MEANS NO RISK OF BREAST CANCER

One of the most common myths about breast cancer has to do with family history. Many women strongly believe that if there is no history of breast cancer or any type of cancer in their family, they can't get breast cancer.

What is true about breast cancer is this: there are many risks associated with breast cancer beyond any genetic or hereditary link. Although we can control some of the risks, there are many risks we are unable to control. There is no single risk or attribute that definitively means you will or will not get breast cancer. Despite years of research, we still do not have a complete understanding of all the ways breast cancer cells begin to develop in the breast.

Women need regular annual screening tests or mammograms to detect any anomalies in the breast tissue and cells. It is even more critical if there is any history of breast cancer in the immediate family.

34. MYTH #2: A LUMP MEANS BREAST CANCER

A lump or knot in your breast does not automatically imply that you have breast cancer. In fact, about 80% of biopsied lumps found in the breast are benign (non-cancerous).[32]

If you find a lump in your breast, you have the option to have it biopsied or have additional diagnostic tests performed. The size and location of the lump will help determine the available testing options. Your doctor will review the options with you and may suggest additional x-rays, an ultrasound, or a biopsy.

Your doctor may also recommend waiting for a few months to see if the shape or size of the lump changes. You always have the right to insist on additional diagnostic tests. Weigh your testing options and understand the potential risks if you choose to wait.[33]

---

[32] Stony Brook Cancer Center (2021). 'Different Kinds of Breast Lumps', *Stony Brook Cancer Center.* Retrieved from https://cancer.stonybrookmedicine.edu/breast-cancer-team/patients/bse/breastlumps.

[33] When I had my first mammogram, I had to go back to St. Luke's Women's Center to get additional tests. I had another mammogram on my right breast, and that second mammogram showed microcalcification, which appeared as a small cluster of dots on the image.

The radiologist explained to me that only 20% of microcalcification clusters turn out to be cancerous. She recommended that I wait for six months and come back for another mammogram to see if the microcalcification cluster had changed in size or shape.

I was not comfortable with waiting for six months with a 20% chance that the cluster of cells was cancerous. I insisted on a biopsy of the area to rule out the presence of cancer. I was fortunate that I made that choice. Four days after my biopsy, I received the news that I had breast cancer. I had elected not to wait for six months before doing additional testing , and I honestly believe that this saved my life.

By the time I went through surgery one month later to remove te breast tissue, the lab tests of that tissue had shown that my cancer was aggressive and had already started to spread. If I had waited six months, it might have already metastasized to other areas of my body.

35. MYTH #3: THE BRCA GENE MUTATION MEANS YOU WILL GET BREAST CANCER

All women have the BRCA1 and BRCA 2 genes, but only about 1 in 500 women have an actual mutation of one of those genes. Even with a mutation, it is not a guarantee that you will develop breast cancer.

If there is a history of breast cancer in your family, you may want to consider genetic testing to determine if you have a BRCA gene mutation. If you do have a mutation, you and your doctor should develop a screening test plan to ensure you are closely monitored for any changes in your breasts.

36. MYTH #4: BREAST CANCER ALWAYS STARTS AS A LUMP

Breast cancer can present itself in a variety of ways. However, many symptoms can be leading indicators of the presence of breast cancer cells, including nipple discharge, skin discoloration, and even dimpling of the breast skin.

Microcalcification is also a potential symptom of breast cancer. However, this is not something you can easily see with the naked eye. Instead, it appears as a bright white dot or cluster of dots somewhere on a breast x-ray. Radiologists have specific training to look for key attributes such as microcalcification and other anomalies that may indicate the presence of cancer cells.

Don't wait to discover a lump before you get regular screening tests. Instead, take your health into your own hands and be proactive with your mammograms.

37. MYTH #5: IF YOU GET BREAST CANCER, YOU WILL DIE

When I first received the news that I had breast cancer, I was utterly devastated. I didn't know what my prognosis was, nor did I have any idea whether or not I would survive. My first thoughts immediately went towards death and dying. I didn't realize how flawed my thinking was until I began to do my own research and learn about my disease, diagnosis, and prognosis.

There are more than 3.8 million women in the United States alone that are breast cancer survivors.[34] I have already shared many reasons why early detection of breast cancer is so important. Many treatments are available, including surgery and chemotherapy that can eliminate cancer cells from the body and help patients live a long and normal life.

---

[34] The American Cancer Society medical and editorial content team (2021). 'How Common Is Breast Cancer', *American Cancer Society.* Retrieved from https://www.cancer.org/cancer/breast-cancer/about/how-common-is-breast-cancer.html.

LIFE WITH BREAST CANCER

38. LIFE WITH BREAST CANCER

When someone is diagnosed with breast cancer, the following weeks, months, and even years of their life will potentially be turned upside down. With the initial diagnosis, there is the emotional struggle of determining which treatment option is best. Each individual has a lot of information to digest before making the final decision on their treatment plan.

Some treatments have minimally visible impacts, such as minor scarring. However, other treatments are much more extreme and can result in large external scars and permanent side effects from chemotherapy and other forms of treatment.

When someone receives a breast cancer diagnosis, it changes them forever. There are psychological effects as well as physical effects. Therefore, it is so essential for anyone diagnosed with breast cancer to find a support person or group that can lift them up and provide an emotional shoulder to lean on during their treatment. Many non-profit organizations have programs and support groups for just that purpose.

If you have been diagnosed with breast cancer, know that you are not alone. You are now part of a

53

pink sisterhood of millions of women who are survivors, many of whom, like myself, strive every day to empower other survivors to express their feelings and talk about concerns with someone who has experienced a similar diagnosis.

As a man with breast cancer, you have many resources available to you, as well. Although not as many men are affected by breast cancer, there is a growing recognition of the risks of male breast cancer in the United States. Many non-profit cancer organizations raise awareness for male breast cancer. One such organization is The Male Breast Cancer Coalition.[35]

If you are supporting someone through a breast cancer diagnosis and treatment, the best thing you can do for them is to "be present." Let that person know you are there to support them emotionally. Give them space to speak freely and share their emotions.

---

[35] The Male Breast Cancer Coalition is an organization that started in 2013. Their mission is to raise awareness of male breast cancer and work towards changing the status quo of the medical community concerning the need for more testing and focused clinical trials for men with breast cancer. You can find out more by visiting their website: https://malebreastcancercoalition.org/.

39. BREAST CANCER: THE SEQUEL

Many movies and films have something referred to as a "sequel hook." The hook is a way the film industry sets up precise openings and possibilities for another story. Although the original story or plot may have closure, some unresolved issues or topics remain open, thus providing a "hook" into a sequel.

A breast cancer diagnosis is very similar to a movie hook. The breast cancer movie timeline starts when you hear the words "you have breast cancer" and ends after your very last treatment for breast cancer disease. At that point, the "movie" ends, but there are still unresolved issues.

The most troubling unresolved issue with any cancer diagnosis and treatment is the inability to guarantee cancer won't return. If you are diagnosed with breast cancer, you will always have a little voice in the back of your mind reminding you that there is a chance, even a small one, that cancer can return. That slight chance may be due to not wholly eradicating every last cancer cell, or it may be the inability to stop the original trigger that caused the cells to change in the first place. Unfortunately, despite numerous hours and countless dollars spent on cancer research, there is still no way to dissipate those open, unresolved issues completely.

The fear of recurrence is an authentic psychological remnant of a cancer diagnosis that every survivor consciously or subconsciously thinks about regularly. The best advice I can give someone who is a friend, a loved one, or a caregiver of a survivor is this: never minimize the fear of a cancer recurrence. It is a reality that we as survivors deal with every single day of our lives. Please support us and encourage us as we learn to deal with and accept the possibility of recurrence.

40. THE FIVE STAGES OF GRIEF

When someone is first diagnosed with breast cancer or any cancer, it is entirely normal and expected that the individual would begin to go through the five stages of grieving. In this section, I want to share my journey through grief with you and the reasoning I went through when I first heard the words "you have breast cancer."

Denial

I immediately asked the question, "Are you sure?" I didn't have a family history of breast cancer, and I didn't feel a lump. How could I have breast cancer? It had to be a mistake.

Anger

Why is this happening to me? I am only 46 years old and still have many years ahead of me for living and enjoying life. What did I do to deserve this? I have done everything right in my life, and I had just lost 40 pounds. I was in the best physical shape I had been in for several years. So why am I the one who has to go through this? I have a strong need to be in control of everything in my life. I was angry that I no longer had control over my health and wellness, and I wanted to lash out at anything and everything that tried to console me, even the people I loved.

Bargaining

God heard a lot from me the first few days after my diagnosis. "I promise I will do better and be better if you just take this cancer away from me." "Just let me get through this now and I will pay it forward later." So many bargaining conversations transpired in those first few days.I bargained and begged and promised so many things that I was incapable of carrying through. It's a good thing he loves unconditionally because I really talked his ear off!

Depression

Depression was something I honestly didn't expect to encounter, but I really hit that stage of grieving pretty hard. Many cancer survivors deal with depression for a very long time after their diagnosis and treatment. It is one of the stages of grieving that tends to stay around for a while. For some people, it never entirely goes away.

I went through the first three stages of grief pretty quickly but then wallowed in self-pity for several days, weeks and months. I was sad. I was still angry. I was still in denial. However, most of all, I couldn't get my mind to stop thinking about whether I would survive. I was also very upset after my double mastectomy. The loss of my breasts was devastating to me, but I talk about that in more detail later on in this book.

When you hear that you have cancer, it is important to surround yourself with people who love and care about you. The support system is extremely critical for your mental health as a cancer patient. Many organizations provide support resources for those who have a strong family and friends support system and for those who don't. Sometimes you just need an outside perspective to help you through the day.

I took advantage of a program that the American Cancer Society offers called "Reach to Recovery."[36] This program pairs you with a cancer survivor in your geographical area (when possible) that has gone through a similar diagnosis and experience as you. They are volunteers who receive training to help another person cope with a breast cancer diagnosis and treatment. The intent is to give you at least one person you can always contact any time of the day or night to help you get through any emotional crisis you may be facing.

Acceptance

Acceptance is the final stage in the grieving process. It does not mean that you are ok with what is happening to you, but you acknowledge that this is your present state. You are accepting that state and no longer trying to change the reality of your current situation.

Acceptance is often challenging to achieve for a cancer survivor. Once you have cancer, you will forever think differently about your life and the lives of those close to you. Cancer has long-term

---

[36] You can find more information about the Reach to Recovery program by visiting their website at https://www.cancer.org/treatment/support-programs-and-services/reach-to-recovery.html.

psychological and emotional effects on a person. The bitterness can last a long time, and the inability to accept the state of your life after cancer is a real thing.

I am fortunate that I had a wonderful support group and came from a long line of strong-spirited ancestors. I was able to rise above my situation and turn it into something positive for me and others. It is also why I am sharing this book with you, my readers.

41. IT'S OK TO MOURN

When I was diagnosed with breast cancer, I was torn over which treatment option was best for me. With several options to choose from, my doctor encouraged me to have a lumpectomy to remove the part of the breast and surrounding tissue infected with cancer cells.

I spent several days mulling over my options. On the one hand, I wanted the easy route with a lumpectomy. If I went that route, I would likely be placed on chemotherapy and radiation to ensure no cancer cells could remain and the infected area of the breast was fully inoculated.

On the other hand, a mastectomy meant removing the entire breast, nipple, areola, and the surrounding fat and tissue. If I chose a mastectomy, radiation would not be required as there would be nothing left to radiate! However, chemotherapy was still a possibility as the doctors wouldn't know the extent of the damage until they cut out the cancer cells. It depended on whether or not the cells had begun to spread within my breast tissue. With a mastectomy, however, I was sacrificing my entire breast. I would have to go through reconstruction. I would no longer have a nipple. I would no longer feel like I was a "complete" woman.

I chose to have a total mastectomy on my right breast and a prophylactic mastectomy on my left breast. I chose to remove the left breast for peace of mind. I wanted to have as little breast tissue left in my body as possible to reduce the risk of any breast cancer recurrence.

The night before my surgery, I literally cried myself to sleep, mourning the pending loss of a part of my body that tends to define our femininity. Surprisingly as I write this, my eyes well up with tears as I remember clearly my emotions, thoughts, and feelings that night.

My boyfriend and I stayed at a hotel close to the hospital the night before my surgery. He was an incredible emotional support for me that night. We spent time talking about what I was about to experience. He allowed me the time to cry and mourn what I was about to lose. He spent time that night caressing me, holding me, and loving me in a very intimate way that I will never forget. It was a final celebration of my natural breasts before the surgeons would remove them the next day.

I knew that my life would be different after this surgery, as would my physical body. I honestly had no idea how much it would affect me, however. Although I do not regret my decision, I wish that I had been more mentally and psychologically prepared for the aftermath of that decision.

I chose to have reconstruction surgery. Yes, I have implants in both breasts now, but I also have angry, red scars where the surgeon opened up each breast to remove all of the breast tissue and fat. The loss of my breasts affected me psychologically much more than I expected. That feminine part of my body is completely gone now, which, as any man or woman knows, actually plays a significant role in any intimate relationship. It took me a long time to even be comfortable being naked in front of my boyfriend, and even to this day, I am still extremely insecure about how my fake breasts look. They are nothing like natural breasts. As long as I have clothes on, you cannot tell that anything is different. My naked body is drastically and forever changed, however.

I still grieve over the loss of my natural breasts, but I am thankful that I am alive and able to share my story with others. I have only started to embrace my scars in the last couple of years. Each day that passes, I realize the importance of the story that those red scars represent. My scars are beautiful and they prove that I am a very strong person and that I conquered cancer. I truly wish every woman could reach a state of peace and security in their physical body after a mastectomy. Still, through my own experience, I know this is just not always a feasible expectation.

42. FLAT FREEDOM

Although I elected to have reconstruction surgery, many women choose to have a mastectomy and **not** have their breast(s) reconstructed. I joined several Facebook support groups right after I was diagnosed with breast cancer. These groups are private and have become a safe haven for me. I was able to post about all my feelings, fears, and insecurities with groups of women who had already experienced similar issues. It was an outlet for me that allowed me to retain some level of sanity throughout my experience.

In one group conversation, I asked for feedback on the things people said or how they were treated differently after their diagnosis and treatment. One lady, Carolyn, explained her story in which she elected not to have her breast reconstructed after she had a total mastectomy. She had reviewed stories from other women who had reconstruction and saw some of the complications they had encountered. She decided she didn't want to deal with any of the potential complications that might come with reconstruction. She didn't want to risk having similar issues.

Carolyn expressed to our private Facebook group that doctors tend to push "fake boobs" on breast cancer survivors. No one seems to talk about what she calls "Flat Freedom". She is now 11 years cancer-free and enjoys the fact that she no longer gets that summer heat rash from wearing a bra!!

Women who choose to go flat after a mastectomy should **never** be ridiculed or have their reasons minimized for choosing to remain flat over going through breast reconstruction. I genuinely believe it is also important for society - every one of us - to recognize, understand, and **know** that breasts do not solely define a woman! Choosing flat freedom goes against everything society expects. However, it is a strong female stance to go against the expectations of how society defines a woman. We are definitely more than our body parts! Thank you, Carolyn, for sharing your experience of flat freedom with me and with others!

HOW TO SUPPORT SOMEONE WITH BREAST CANCER

43. SUPPORTING SOMEONE WITH BREAST CANCER

On Tuesday, June 23rd, 2015, at 10:00 am, I received a call from St. Luke's Women's Center in Chesterfield, Missouri. That single phone call and the conversation changed my life forever. That morning I heard the words, "you have breast cancer."

I was in shock. This wasn't happening, especially not to me. I felt fine and, in fact, was in the best physical shape I had been in for years. I had been exercising and eating healthy and had lost almost 40 pounds over the previous 12 months. They must have made a mistake and switched my results with someone else. There was no other explanation.

In my heart, however, I knew this wasn't true. I had breast cancer and had to deal with it. I didn't want to die. I didn't want to lose my hair. I didn't want to go through chemotherapy. I didn't want to deal with this at all. I wanted to crawl into a corner, curl up in a fetal position, and just pretend like I was invisible. But I had to face this curveball life had thrown my way. I either needed to catch it or let it run me over. I had a choice to make.

Many women and men go through a roller coaster of emotions when informed they have breast cancer. It is incredibly difficult to process those four words. Individually, they are words that do not amount to anything special. However, when you put those words together, those words change your life forever: **<u>You have breast cancer.</u>**

Each of us probably knows someone who has been affected by breast cancer. After experiencing the breast cancer journey myself, I have many insights into how you can support a friend or loved one facing a breast cancer diagnosis.

44. THINGS TO NEVER SAY

As human beings, most of us try to be empathetic when we learn that someone is dealing with an illness, disease, or even death in the family. Most of us want to provide positive "help" to someone who is dealing with a tragedy.

As friends, family,and co-workers began to learn about my breast cancer diagnosis, I was shocked to hear how those same individuals decided to "help" me through their words. No one intended for their comments to be malicious or insensitive. On the contrary, I'm sure people made all the comments with heartfelt good intentions. The outcome, in some cases, however, was not always a positive or helpful one for me.

Here are some examples of phrases that I received from people trying to "help" me:

"You're so lucky because now you get a free boob job."

Contrary to what it might seem, having a mastectomy with reconstruction isn't as glamorous as it may sound. Reconstruction is **not** anything close to a breast augmentation or reduction surgery. It is also important to recognize that many women who have a mastectomy do not have the ability to save the nipple and areola. Just think about what that means in relation to a "free boob job". They are not in the same category at all.

I had to have two breast reconstruction surgeries. During my double mastectomy surgery in July of 2015, the surgeon inserted expanders beneath my chest muscles in each breast. Over the next few months, I had to go to the doctor for several appointments to have a saline solution injected into each expander. The purpose of this was to gradually stretch the breast tissue and muscle to make room for inserting the implants later.

In December of 2015, I had my "exchange" surgery. During this surgery, the surgeon removes the fully injected expanders and replaces them with actual implants. Within about eight months, however, the surgery failed. My implants moved out from under the chest muscles and pushed out towards the outside of my chest area. Now I required a second reconstruction surgery to fix the issues caused by the failed first surgery. With this second surgery, the surgeon placed the implants on top of the muscles, but they still did not hold up too well. When you have a mastectomy, the surgical process destroys most of the structure and foundation of the breast. As a result, I have very little in my chest area that can hold implants in place. After a mastectomy, the lack of breast structure is a common challenge with women who have breast reconstruction.

Although I now have "foobs" (fake boobs), they are not the same as breasts that still have natural breast tissue augmented with additional implants or fat grafting. In other words, it wasn't a free boob job.

"My grandmother (or uncle, or cousin, or friend) had cancer, but they died …."

Right after my diagnosis, my primary focus was figuring out how to **live**. I have had relatives die from cancer. So I already know it's a possibility. It's just not something I wanted to face when I still had no guarantee that I was even going to survive this! I did not and do not wish to be reminded that people still die from cancer.

"You look so healthy! Are you sure it's cancer?"

Typically, when cancer is first detected, the individual with cancer will appear to be perfectly healthy. However, once treatment begins, side effects and other complications can affect the individual's appearance and health.

Questioning the diagnosis only creates additional doubt in someone's mind. Believe me when I say there is already plenty of doubt to go around. Every day, I questioned whether or not this was truly real and happening to me. I wanted to believe in the doubt, but believing in that would mean a delay in dealing with the significant issue at hand. I was fighting for my life.

"My friend tried this natural treatment that cured her cancer ...."

When a doctor recommends a cancer treatment, they design the treatment to be very specific for that individual. What works for one person may very well

71

not work for another person, even if the types of cancer are exactly the same. For this reason, researchers continue to look towards individualized treatments. For example, chemotherapy is now more of a cocktail of medicines designed and integrated together to attack an individual's own cancer specifically. The chemotherapy regimen for one person will very likely be different from someone else that has the exact same type of cancer.

"That's a good kind of cancer to have ...."

I will keep this rebuttal short and sweet. There is no good kind of cancer. Cancer is a horrible disease that no one should ever have to go through.

"I know how you feel."

At a very early age in my life, I learned that I could never know exactly how someone else feels about anything. Now, do I still say this sometimes? Yes, it does naturally slip out occasionally. However, if someone has breast cancer, and you have never had it, please do not ever tell them you know how they feel. You don't, and you can't.

My breast cancer experience and how I dealt with it will be much different from how another survivor thinks about their own breast cancer experience. Find other ways to empathize and share your support with your friend or loved one. They want to know you support them. If you have never dealt with a cancer diagnosis personally, you have no clue how I am feeling.

45. WHAT TO SAY TO SOMEONE WITH BREAST CANCER

The best answer I have ever gotten from someone regarding my breast cancer diagnosis was this: "I don't know what to say."

It's ok not to know what to say. When I first heard I had breast cancer, I didn't even know what to express myself. There is nothing you really can say. Just be there and support your friend or loved one. They need to know that you care and that you are supportive of them.

You can also say something like, "I'm sorry (or sad) that you are going through this." Acknowledging that the situation is crappy goes a long way.

I want to get this main point across to you: Think about what you are saying before saying it. This is true for anything in life, but when it comes to helping someone cope with a cancer diagnosis, think before speaking. Ensure you are not getting ready to say something so insensitive that it causes a setback for the person with the diagnosis.

46. ASK THE QUESTION: HOW CAN I HELP

As a friend or supporter of someone with cancer, one of the hardest things to do is admit that you cannot fix the problem. This doesn't mean that you cannot help them or be useful, however. Instead of assuming you know what your friend or loved one needs, it's always better to ask them. However, keep in mind that most of us are very proud people, and never like to admit we need help.

When I was recovering from my double mastectomy surgery, my friends asked what I needed. My initial response was "nothing." I didn't want to look weak or appear as if I couldn't take care of myself. Responding with "nothing" isn't necessarily the best approach, however.

My brother once told me something that has stayed with me to this day. If you are an outsider looking in and want to help someone through a traumatic experience, it's a two-way street. As the person dealing with a breast cancer diagnosis and surgery, I needed to put aside my pride as the "victim" of the traumatic experience. Other people need to feel valuable and helpful in a time of crisis. It is their way of giving back to me and showing support in a situation where they have no control whatsoever. I needed to allow them to have some control and to be able to participate in my recovery. I encourage anyone who is dealing with a breast cancer diagnosis and treatment to do the same thing! Let others help you!

47. BE STILL AND LISTEN

As I was recovering from my first surgery, I had a lot of time just lying around, not being able to do anything at all. I felt so helpless. It took everything I had in me not to slip into a state of constant depression and negativity.

I had a couple of very close friends and family members that recognized I sometimes just needed to talk. One of the most lovely things you can do for someone with cancer is to "be present" with them. Listen to what they are saying. Could you encourage them to discuss their fears? Help them work through the anxiety that comes with every sharp pain and every out-of-place or abnormal symptom. Just listen. Sometimes that is the best gift anyone can provide.

48. CARE PACKAGES AND ENCOURAGEMENT

I have some very dear friends who dropped off a care package for me during the recovery period after my first surgery. The care package had all kinds of thoughtful items to help me pass the time. A care package is one of the most endearing and caring ways to show someone you are thinking about them. As someone dealing with the aftermath of a double mastectomy, the biggest thing I really needed was distractions. Otherwise, I would begin that downward spiral towards depression and sadness. My overactive imagination filled my thoughts with the grief and despair of losing a part of my femininity.

It's important to note that it is often challenging to focus on anything requiring cognitive thinking after surgery or a chemotherapy cycle. I wanted to watch TV all day or listen to music. I am an avid reader, but I couldn't read more than a page before I quickly became tired and lost interest. Any items you include in a care package should consider these challenges!

There are many great ideas for items to include in a care package (aside from food or snacks). Here are a few suggestions:

- Word search books
- Adult coloring books and colored pencils
- Warm blanket
- Warm socks
- Fancy water bottle (with bling!)
- Audiobooks
- Inspirational quotes

My co-workers sent me balloons with hand-written "get well" and "thinking of you" cards attached to them. I read every single one of them and left the balloons and cards floating in my living room every day, so I could see them while I was watching TV or falling asleep. When the balloons lost their air, I detached the cards and hung them up on my fireplace mantel. I left those notes up there for months. It helped me through some of my more challenging and woe-is-me moments and gave me the courage to keep moving forward every day. I still have those cards tucked away in a small box in my office at home.

Years ago, I had a friend (former co-worker) going through a difficult time separating from his wife. At that time, I wrote him a quick note every day while he was going through his experience. My intention for that single daily note was to give him a spark of hope and a glimpse of positivity to keep his spirits high and in check for that day. In this digital age, even sending a quick text message every day or every other day goes a long way. Don't underestimate the importance of sending a "Thinking of you" or "Hugs" text for someone who has been diagnosed with breast cancer or is recovering from surgery.

In 2015, my work family at Nestle Purina did the most fantastic thing imaginable when I was recovering at home from my surgery. Every Friday, they would gather in the lobby of our building and have someone on the 2nd-floor balcony take a picture of them. They would position themselves with pink flowy fabric in the shape of a cancer ribbon, and every single person would wear something pink to represent their support and awareness of breast cancer. There were pink hats, pink shoes, pink shirts and even pink hair. Every Friday, I would get that picture, and it gave me something to look forward to and carried me through the long weekend. It was incredibly humbling to know that so many people cared about me and what I was going through.

I will never forget those pictures or that gesture of encouragement from that team. They gave me the strength to carry forward even when I was so tired and weak that I didn't want to move on anymore. I know I sent thank you cards, but that work-family will probably never know how much those seemingly little acts of kindness meant to me. They truly gave me hope and courage to keep pushing my way through my recovery.

49. HOME COOKED MEALS VERSUS GIFT CARDS

I sat and watched TV all day when I was recovering from my surgery, and I usually ended up falling asleep just a few minutes into the show. During this time, the last thing I wanted to do was think about cooking.

I had wonderful friends who put together a meal calendar for my boyfriend and me. We had meals delivered to our house by a food delivery service, or friends would drop off homemade food at our home during their lunch break. We had so many excellent meals and desserts - I was truly blessed and fortunate to have so many people that cared about me.

I had a couple of friends who sent me some gift cards in the mail that were good for local restaurants in my area. Those were perfect, as well, because we could call ahead for some take-out food, and my boyfriend could go pick up the food and bring it back home for us.

Everyone needs to eat, right? Gift cards or food delivery is one of the most straightforward and thoughtful things you can do for someone recovering from surgery!

50. DON'T WAIT TO BE ASKED

I am a very proud and independent person, and I have always had difficulty asking anyone for help. I suspect many women and men have the same struggle as I do. If you have a friend or a loved one going through a breast cancer diagnosis or recovering from surgery, do them a huge favor. Offer to do something for them, and tell them they cannot refuse you!

Tell your friend you will be bringing dinner to their home next week, or offer to take them to their next doctor appointment. Find out if they have a salon and take them there to get their hair washed and styled. After my surgery, I couldn't wash my hair on my own for almost three weeks because I couldn't raise my arms that high. Talk about misery!

Be open with your friend or loved one and ask what they need. If the response is "nothing", don't accept it. Ask again until you get a response you can act on and an answer you need!

If you want to support someone going through breast cancer, go all in. Don't stop at just being present. Do things for them that you know they are unable to do for themselves. Pamper them, console them, and let them know you care. The acts of kindness that we show to others are precious. It's the gift that keeps on giving. It's something we should all do in life always with no questions asked.

After reading this book, I hope you better understand what life can be like for someone with breast cancer. No one should ever face a breast cancer diagnosis or treatment alone. If you have the chance, be present for someone who is facing breast cancer. Pay it forward. You may be surprised at how wonderful it feels to know you are helping someone through an incredibly emotional and physically draining time in their life. Show them love, compassion, and empathy. Be present.

OTHER HELPFUL RESOURCES

American Cancer Society: https://www.cancer.org/

BreastCancer.org: https://www.breastcancer.org/

Centers For Disease Control - Screening for Breast Cancer: https://www.cdc.gov/cancer/breast/basic_info/screening.htm

National Cancer Institute: https://www.cancer.gov/

READ OTHER
50 THINGS TO KNOW
BOOKS

50 Things to Know

Stay up to date with new releases on Amazon:
https://amzn.to/2VPNGr7

CZYKPublishing.com

50 Things to Know

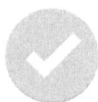

We'd love to hear what you think about our content! Please leave your honest review of this book on Amazon and Goodreads. We appreciate your positive and constructive feedback. Thank you.

Printed in Great Britain
by Amazon

82891520R00058